The Curl C[...]s Guide

"Perfect for every natural girl"

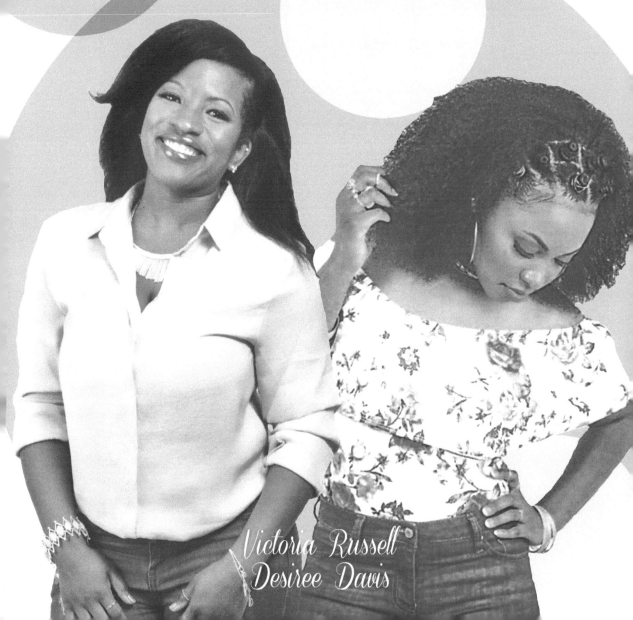

Victoria Russell
Desiree Davis

Outskirts Press, Inc.
http://www.outskirtspress.com

ISBN: 978-1-4787-9179-9

Outskirts Press and the "OP" logo are trademarks belonging to Outskirts Press, Inc.

PRINTED IN THE UNITED STATES OF AMERICA

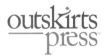

Disclaimer

The contents of this guide are strictly what has worked for us. We are not hair experts of any kind. We have learned through trial and error and found things that have worked for us. Our goal is to share that information with you. We hope that each and every one of you are able to take something from this guide and use it to help you in your natural hair journey. We continue to learn new things every day. As we learn more, we will continue to share.

Table of Contents

Introduction:
So You Want to Go Natural

So you want to go natural? You want to grow long and healthy hair? We put this guide together just for you. Back when we first started our natural hair journey there weren't nearly as many resources as there are now. Today, there is a huge selection of products for naturals. Most hair care companies have a special line of products for natural girls. There's even products for girls who are transitioning.

This guide will cover all the things that we wish we would have known years ago when we first started our natural hair journey. We will speak from experience as well as some research. We hope this guide will help you avoid the pitfalls we experienced.

Desiree and I have different hair textures, we went natural in different ways and we ultimately have different styling routines. So this guide is perfect for just about every natural girl. Are you the natural that wants to rock a wash and go? Desiree has all the tips you need to have those curls pop in no time. Do you love protective styles like buns, braids, twists, wigs and weaves? Well that's where I come in. We joined together to bring you ladies an all in one guide to growing long natural hair!

WHY DID WE DECIDE TO GO NATURAL?

Desiree

When I was in college, I got tired of wearing the same hairstyle I had since high school. I was sick of wearing the same flat look and it never growing. One day I decided I wanted to do something new with my hair so I relaxed it and bleached it two weeks later even though my beautician told me it wasn't a good idea. My hair instantly started falling out and I had to figure it out quickly. I always had a ton of hair but I didn't always know how to manage it and now I was really lost. Right around that time the natural hair movement began and I started seeing girls pop up with curly hair. I wanted that! Long story short, I got the courage to chop all my hair off. I've been natural ever since. I figured short hair was easier to manage.

Victoria

Honestly, I just wanted long hair. Relaxers and chemicals made it hard to retain length. I just couldn't grow my relaxed hair past a certain length. I experienced some major breakage from a certain hair product and that was the last straw for me. I decided to be relaxer free. I wanted a full head of hair. I didn't want to have to wear weave just to have hair down my back. I wanted to prove to myself and the people around me that black girls can have long hair without being "mixed" or wearing weave. It was a journey that was well worth it.

Now that you know a little more about our story, let's help you create your own hair growth story.

CHAPTER 1

To Big Chop or Transition

When it comes to going natural you can either big chop or transition. Both have some benefits and drawbacks. Both will lead you to a head full of natural long hair if you take care of your hair as it grows.

Desiree and I both chose different paths to going natural. Desiree decided to big chop (she actually big chopped twice!) and I decided to transition (I cut my relaxed hair off after about a year of transitioning). So we'll go over both topics from experience.

The biggest thing to remember is to choose what ultimately will work for you.

So I'll kick things off with giving you the lowdown on transitioning.

TRANSITIONING

Let's be honest. The idea of chopping off all of your hair at one time is terrifying. Especially because I was obsessed with having long hair all my life. Even if I knew the hair would eventually grow back, I still didn't want short hair. I'd get mad if a stylist even trimmed too much of my hair off. I knew I could not big chop. I refused to walk around bald headed or with a short fro. Although some women pull it off quite well. I was terrified of the "ugly/awkward stage". I knew I wanted to go natural, but I wanted to do it my way. Slowly.

Transitioning seemed a lot better for me because I could change my mind at any time and go back to relaxing my hair. Transitioning was like a long test drive before officially hopping on the natural bandwagon.

Going natural was a big decision and I knew nothing about it. What if my texture wasn't like the girls I saw on YouTube? What if I hated being natural? What if my hair still didn't grow as long as I wanted it to? These were all questions I had. Before I get into how to transition, let me give you my transitioning story.

My Transitioning Story

After I had some major hair breakage, I decided that I had to rid my hair of the harsh chemicals in relaxers. The middle section of my hair broke off really bad. I was tired of wearing weave and my real hair was in bad shape. I noticed Desiree had went natural and her hair was so beautiful and full. Her hair literally had grown overnight. She convinced me it was worth going natural.

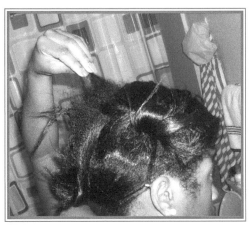

I didn't really set a deadline for how long I would transition. After I transitioned for about a year, one day I got so tired of dealing with two textures I decided to cut off the rest of my relaxed hair. I was wearing wigs all the time so no one would really know I had cut my hair.

For almost 2 years I did not show my real hair. I was not comfortable with it and I was still learning how to manage it. I wore tons of full sew in weaves, box braids and wigs. At first my natural hair texture was dry and frizzy. I didn't see any defined curl pattern in sight. With a lot of patience and moisturizing, my curls finally started to come through.

From my transitioning experience, here's some tips to avoid my pitfalls:

- **Do** deep condition weekly if possible.
- **Do** comb from the ends of your hair to the root with a **wide** tooth comb.
- **Do** take breaks in between protective styling to avoid putting too much tension on your hair.
- **Do** take the time to play with and learn your texture.
- **Do** wear protective styles but styles that allow you to moisturize your hair as often as possible.
- **Do** make sure you start using natural hair products.

- **Don't** comb your hair too much.
- **Do** be careful where your natural hair meets your relaxed hair (line of demarcation)—it's very fragile.
- **Do** set a timeline for you to cut off your relaxed hair.
- **Do** find a style that works for you.
- **Don't** go out and buy too many products too soon, keep it simple.
- **Do** use YouTube.
- **Do** understand shrinkage is not bad, it can be annoying but definitely not a bad thing.
- **Do** start washing your hair in sections, this will save you as your hair gets longer and it will make wash day so much easier.
- **Don't** straighten your hair too much trying to get your natural texture to blend with your relaxed texture.
- **Don't** hold on to your relaxed ends too long.
- **Don't** wash your hair without detangling first.

Tip: Herbal Essence Hello Hydration Moisturizing Conditioner and Aussie Moist Conditioners are great cheap conditioners to detangle your hair.

PROS VS CONS OF TRANSITIONING

Pros:

- You get to keep your length—when you big chop you are starting from scratch.
- You have the option of changing your mind and going back to a relaxer. (I doubt you will!)
- It's a slow gradual change into the natural world.

Cons:

- Hair is extremely fragile where the two textures meet so it requires a lot of patience.
- Natural styles don't work as effortlessly because your relaxed ends are straight when the rest of your hair is curly.
- Some naturals will try to convince you to big chop before you are ready and some relaxed girls will try to talk you out of going natural.

BIG CHOP

Since Victoria gave you the lowdown on transitioning, I guess it would make sense for me to explain my big chop experience. It seemed like going natural became a big sensation overnight. I was in the middle of trying to figure out what to do with my damaged hair and I was getting impatient. I knew nothing about transitioning so doing a big chop seemed like the only option for me. I never had short hair before and I was honestly terrified of having a short fro but I wasn't going to let that stop me.

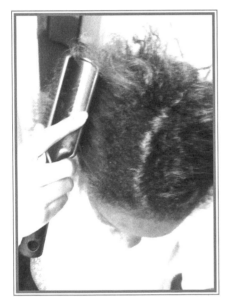

Doing a big chop was as easy as cutting all my hair off. Why did I feel like it was so much deeper? I had been with this hair all my life and never imagined cutting it off. I knew that if I decided to cut my hair off there was no going back. But I was done with my hair and I had a decision to make.

At the time when I decided to go natural, the only thing I thought about was all the beautiful curls I had seen. Nobody really talked about transitioning so it was either big chop or stick with the "creamy crack". I always had what you considered "good hair" so I wasn't concerned with what my curl pattern would be like. My only concern was not feeling comfortable in my own skin and having to resort to braids or wigs. Let me give you my big chop story.

My Big Chop Story

Let's just say your stylist isn't lying when they say that bleaching your hair takes it to a whole other level. It can and will break your hair off if you don't take care of it. Truth is I never took great care of my hair prior to coloring it. Against the advice of my stylist, I bleached my hair. My hair started breaking off in the front first and before I knew it my hair was breaking off all over. I went into panic mode.

I knew I wanted to big chop but I was scared of having a fro, so I got it cut into a mohawk. A few days later I didn't like the look so I chopped some more hair off and left myself a long bang. When my natural hair texture started growing in I loved my curls. The only problem was that it didn't match my straight, relaxed hair. I decided it was time for those relaxed ends to go. My fro fear came to life and I started throwing weave and braids in back to back.

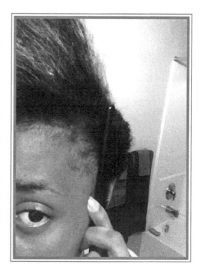

About a year later my hair had finally grown enough to get me out of the "ugly/awkward stage" and I began to embrace my hair. My curl pattern wasn't fully there yet, but it was cute enough to wear in a fro-hawk and that is exactly what I did. Over the next few years YouTube became my best friend and I tried many products, but I never really mastered the art of caring for my hair. My hair grew to about my bra strap by 2016 and all of a sudden it seemed like it stopped growing. I had stopped taking care of my hair, my stress levels were high, and my hair was severely dry. My ends were splitting too fast and my hair got shorter. I could not stop the breakage. I didn't have the money to go to a salon every week and let them take care of it. The thought of my hair falling out stressed me out even more.

Fast forward to November of 2016, I got the urge to just cut it off again. I had gone through a bad breakup and I felt like my hair was holding all that stress and I wanted it gone. I texted Victoria one Saturday and said "I'm coming in town. Can you cut my hair please!". She was very reluctant, but she carried out my wish. The minute she cut it I got depressed and regretted my decision. I felt like I looked like a boy and once again I didn't have a curl pattern. I tried wigs and braids once again but it didn't change a thing. I made the decision to cut my hair and I was going to have to embrace it. With Victoria's help and the discovery of the right hair products for my hair type, I finally got it right and my hair is growing healthier and faster than ever!

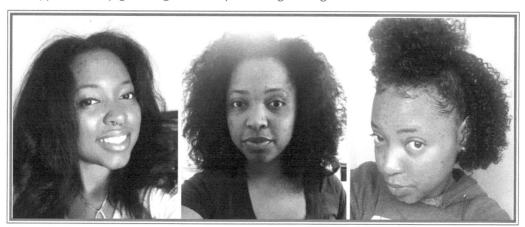

From my big chop experience, here's some tips to help you successfully big chop and be on your way to long hair:

- **Do** make sure you are ready to cut your hair. Chop a few inches and see how you feel. Then go back and chop a few more.
- **Do** deep condition weekly to hydrate your newly forming curls.
- **Do** discover your hair type and porosity so that you can find the best products for your hair. The sooner the better!
- **Don't** let the opinions of others ruin your experience.
- **Do** stay away from heat. Too much heat is very drying and damaging to your hair which can prevent your hair from growing to its maximum potential.
- **Do** understand that your curl pattern and amount of shrinkage you have will be different from other naturals.
- **Do** use a good detangler and comb from the ends to the roots to avoid breakage.
- **Don't** be afraid of short hair. It is just hair and it will grow back.
- **Do** wear a bonnet at night to keep your hair from drying out.
- **Do** use cute accessories to dress yourself up.

PROS VS CONS OF BIG CHOP

Pros:

- Teaches you to embrace your inner beauty.
- It forces you to completely commit to being natural without holding on to your relaxed hair.
- Easier to style and maintain your hair since you are not fighting two textures.

Cons:

- Have to adjust to short hair and there aren't many ways to style it.
- May not have a curl pattern immediately, it takes time to grow in.
- Negative attitudes and judgement from others.

Tip: If you are ready to big chop, head over to YouTube and watch a few tutorials before you give it a try.

CHAPTER 2

The Goddess Guide to Building a Hair Regimen

Building a hair regimen is all about preparation and planning. It takes a lot of trial and error but this chapter is going to make it a lot easier for you to build your very own hair regimen. We'll cover all the topics listed below:

- Hair Porosity
- Hair Regimen Basics
- Heat vs. No Heat
- Winter Hair Care vs. Summer Hair Care
- Charting Your Hair Growth

A hair regimen is your plan and your routine that will make growing your natural hair so much easier. Trust us. It will work wonders for your hair. We will cover each topic starting with hair porosity.

HAIR POROSITY

Without getting too complicated, let's talk about hair porosity. In simple terms, it's your hair's ability to absorb and retain moisture.

Why should you care about it? Retaining hair length is all about keeping your hair moisturized (especially those ends). Knowing your hair porosity will help you figure out how to get moisture into your hair and help it stay there. It'll save you a ton of money because you will know what type of products are good for your hair instead of buying and guessing.

So how do you figure out your hair's porosity? You can do a strand test by following the below steps:

- Take a few strands of freshly washed hair.
- Put it in a bowl of room temperature water.
- Watch it for a few minutes to see if the hair floats, sinks right away or slowly sinks.
- If your hair sinks right away you have **high porosity**, if it floats you have **low porosity** and if it sinks slowly you have **medium** or **normal porosity.**

Side Note: I find many naturals have low porosity hair, which may explain why so many naturals complain about having dry hair. Low porosity hair has the most trouble getting moisture into the hair.

Here's what you need to know about **low porosity hair**.

Characteristics

- Tight cuticle
- Hard to get moisture in or out of the hair
- Susceptible to product build up
- Doesn't need heavy products
- Longer drying time

Tips

- Use lighter products and oils.
- Deep condition with heat to open your hair cuticle—a hair steamer is a great option.
- Find products that contain humectants (honey, vegetable glycerin, etc).
- Invest in a quality clarifying shampoo to remove product buildup .
- Only do a protein treatment if your hair really needs it.
- Try LCO method instead of LOC method (If you do not know anything about the LOC method, research it and it's many benefits).
- Rinse your deep conditioner out with warm water to keep your hair cuticle open before applying your leave-in conditioner.

Oils Perfect for Low Porosity Hair

- Grapeseed Oil
- Jojoba Oil
- Argan Oil
- Sweet Almond Oil

High porosity hair is a little different. With high porosity hair, getting moisture into the hair is not difficult. Getting moisture to stay in the hair is the issue.

Characteristics

- Cuticle is raised/open
- Quickly absorbs moisture but loses it just as quickly
- Can absorb too much moisture
- Hair may be damaged due to use of chemicals or too much heat
- Tangles easily due to raised cuticle

Tips

- Add a protein treatment to your regimen
- Use thick oils/butters to seal in the moisture

Oils Perfect for High Porosity Hair

- Castor oil
- Coconut Oil

Normal porosity needs no deep explanation. Your hair absorbs the right amount of moisture.

HAIR REGIMEN BASICS

Now that we've covered some of the basics about natural hair, it's time to move on to creating your very own hair regimen. We get tons of questions about how we grew our hair and the truth is that the secret to growing long hair is all about preparation and planning.

Some people are blessed with awesome genetics that allow their hair to grow long without them ever having to try. We all know someone who has hair that seems to grow overnight. Unfortunately, some of us have to work for every inch of length and fight to keep it from breaking.

A **hair regimen** is basically your very own hair diet. We all know how annoying diets can be.

But **IF** you stick to your "hair diet", you will reap the benefits of long, moisturized and healthy hair.

Where do I start?

1. Set your hair goal.
2. Find your hair porosity.
3. Figure out the current state of your hair.
4. Get a notebook out and take notes!

Basics for Building a Regimen

+ Write down all the products you already have and rate them. I keep a running list of every product I have ever tried and if I liked it or not. (There are a special set of pages at the end of this guide just for this step!)
+ Decide what products you need to change and what products you are missing.
+ Experiment until you find what works for you.
+ Don't go out and buy too many new products at once.
+ Listen to your hair & don't ignore signs of dry or damaged hair.

Components of a Regimen

To keep it as simple and to the point as possible below is what I suggest you incorporate into your hair regimen. I'll cover each component in detail.

+ Cleanse
+ Condition
+ Moisturize
+ Style

Cleanse

You will see and hear various ways that naturals cleanse their hair. Some will tell you that they never use shampoo and that they only cowash their hair. Some have embraced the "curly girl method" and have had great results. Other natural girls are firm believers in the need for a weekly shampoo.

In my opinion, I think a good cleanse with shampoo is beneficial to the hair every once in awhile. How often you need to cleanse is based on your lifestyle.

Cowash vs. Shampoo

Cowashing is basically washing your hair with a conditioner. It's perfect for softening and refreshing your hair with moisture.

Washing the hair with shampoo is all about cleansing the hair. Look for a good shampoo without sulfates. These shampoos will gently cleanse your hair without stripping your hair too much of its natural oils.

I will say that I do use a sulfate shampoo before I straighten my hair. We'll cover the importance of flat ironing freshly washed hair later.

Clarifying Shampoo vs. Moisturizing Shampoo

A **clarifying shampoo** is great for getting rid of all the product buildup. Many naturals use styling products and over time all that product buildup is left on your hair. A clarifying shampoo will remove that buildup.

On the other hand, a **moisturizing shampoo** has ingredients that are more moisturizing to your hair while cleansing the hair.

You can find a list of our favorite shampoos in Chapter 7.

Tips for wash day:

1. Wash your hair in sections.
2. Massage your scalp softly.
3. Rotate shampoos—I try to keep two different shampoos in my collection.
4. Treat wash day like a spa day and enjoy pampering your hair.

Condition

Conditioning is probably the single most important part of your regimen. There are several types of conditioners and it's important to know the difference. If you do the conditioning step right, your curls will be detangled and hydrated. You will start to see those curls pop in no time.

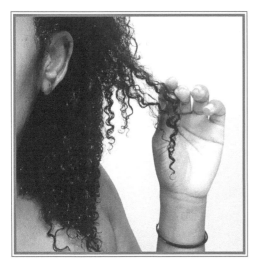

Your hair's best friend is a **deep conditioner.** These conditioners have ingredients that pack serious moisture for your hair. If you see a conditioner that says to leave it in for 15 minutes or longer, chances are it's a deep conditioner. We have a list of those in Chapter 7 too. Deep conditioning with heat will open up your hair cuticle to help the moisture really get deep into your hair. I deep condition every wash and I wash my hair weekly unless I have braids or some other protective style in. Every time I shampoo, I follow up with a deep conditioner. Remember that when you cleanse your hair you are stripping it of its natural oils. It's important to put moisture back into the hair.

Next, you have **cowash conditioners**. These conditioners are often cheap conditioners that may tell you to leave it in for a few minutes. I use these when I cowash my hair. This is also moisturizing to your hair and will help you keep your curls soft and detangled.

Protein conditioners or protein treatments are meant to strengthen the hair. It's easy to overdo these treatments or use them incorrectly and end up with dry, hard hair. Personally, I only do a protein treatment if my hair seems brittle and weak. If you're not sure if you need a protein treatment, try a mild one and see if your hair feels any different after. If you are going to use a protein treatment make sure you follow up with a moisturizing conditioner to add softness back to the hair.

Lastly, we have **leave-in conditioners.** These are extremely important. This can be a liquid or a cream based conditioner. This provides your hair with moisture that will stay in your hair. These conditioners should have water listed as one of the first ingredients. Many natural girls like creamy leave-in conditioners but I have tried some liquid leave-in conditioners that work wonders as well.

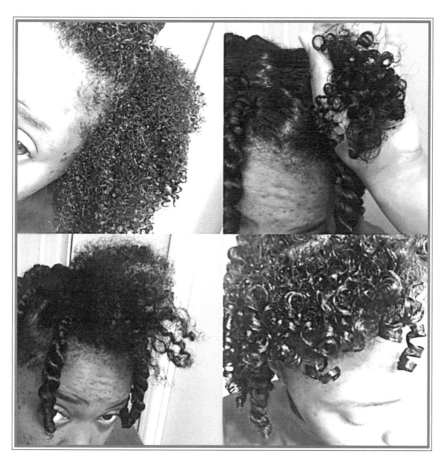

Courtesy of: Mielle Organics White Peony Leave-In Conditioner

Moisturize

So this step should be done daily or every few days if you really want to grow long hair. I moisturize my hair daily. Sometimes I get lazy and miss a day or two but it's important to moisturize your hair daily.

When should you moisturize?

I like to do my moisturizing at night right before bed. I get better results when I moisturize, put on a scarf and let it penetrate my hair overnight without the outside elements getting to it. The next morning all I need to do is style my hair.

What to look for in a good moisturizer?

Look for water to be in the first few ingredients. Water is the best moisturizer so you want a good daily moisturizer that has water as one of its main ingredients. I have had excellent results using my leave-in conditioner as my daily moisturizer.

How do I moisturize?

1. Part my hair in 4 sections.
2. Apply leave-in conditioner to each section.
3. Apply my homemade whipped shea butter on top.
4. Seal it in with a small amount of jojoba oil.

I don't comb my hair unless needed and I never comb my natural hair when it's dry. I save all my detangling for wash day. This allows me to manipulate my hair less. Less manipulation allows your hair to grow in peace.

We can't forget about scalp care. Your scalp produces it's own natural oil, but some naturals still suffer from dry scalp. I apply a very small amount of oil to my scalp about once or twice a week. You don't want to clog your pores so I would go light on the oil. Instead give yourself a scalp massage and allow your hair's natural oils to work.

Most naturals have heard of the LOC method or the LCO method. This method involves applying your products in a certain order to maximize moisture. Google or YouTube it and see if it is something that may work for you. I have personally been doing it for some years and it has done wonders for my hair.

Style

So the fun part about being natural is styling your beautiful hair. There are a million styles that naturals can do. **Versatility** is one of the greatest perks of being natural and don't let anyone tell you any different.

Personally, I don't use too many styling products. Most of my looks can be created just by doing my moisturizing routine and twisting or braiding my hair overnight.

If you do use a styling product and experience flakiness, it may be due to the combination of products you are using. Some products don't mix well. Experiment. See what works for you. The fun part is trying and failing and trying again until you finally find something that works.

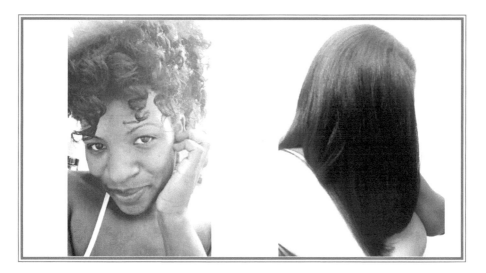

Tip: Be sure to wrap your hair every night in a satin or silk scarf or bonnet.

So now that you know what should go into your regimen, the next question is how often should you use each product. Honestly, that differs for everyone. For example, if you workout five days a week, you probably will need to cleanse your hair more than someone who does not work out. The best advice is to experiment and see what works for your hair and lifestyle.

Wash Day

You will hear us use the term "wash day" throughout this book. Most naturals tend to dedicate a day as their "wash day". For me this tends to be Saturdays. I spend all day cleaning and doing errands around the house while letting my pre-poo or conditioner sit in my hair.

My wash day tends to start the night before. I often apply an oil to my hair and scalp and sleep in it overnight. This is my "prepoo". Desiree and I will share each of our wash day routines in this chapter as well.

First, it's important to understand why wash day is so crucial to a healthy hair journey.

- It preps your hair for styles
- It moisturizes your hair
- It helps with hair repair
- It is one of the only times I comb/detangle my hair

Victoria's Typical Wash Day

1. Pre-poo my hair with olive oil, coconut oil or a mix of oils for an hour or overnight.
2. Shampoo or cowash my hair in 4 sections and thoroughly detangle my hair.
3. Apply my deep conditioner in 4 sections and comb it through. Cover my hair with a plastic cap and a hot towel for about an hour or sit under a hooded dryer for 15-30 minutes.
4. Rinse hair and proceed to apply my leave-in, whipped shea butter and a light oil.
5. Put hair in 8 big twists to air dry before styling.

Desiree's Typical Wash Day

1. Pre-poo with water/aloe vera mix and coconut oil for an hour or overnight.
2. Part hair into 4 sections and apply shampoo or cowash to the scalp of each section first, then the tips.
3. Rinse sections and apply deep conditioner while finger detangling. Deep condition for 30 minutes with a plastic cap under a hooded dryer.
4. Rinse my hair and LCO.
5. Style!

HEAT VS. NO HEAT

Growing up black you were no stranger to a hot comb and flat iron on a regular basis. Along with relaxers, these tools were used to control and maintain your thick hair. Our mothers, aunts and beauticians thought they were doing the best for our hair. Most of them didn't realize they were applying too much heat to our tresses. Not to mention the fact that most of us had relaxers to begin with. Majority of us carried those habits into adulthood which was killing our hair. We are here to tell you to drop those heat habits if you want to see maximum growth!

What are some common heat methods?

- Blow Dryer
- Hooded Dryer
- Flat Iron
- Pressing Comb
- Curling Iron
- Diffuser
- Wand Curler

Depending on which method of heat you are using, here are some tips to keep in mind.

Blow Dryer:

- Blow dry your hair about 75% dry and let it air-dry the rest of the way to reduce moisture depletion.
- Keep blow dryer on medium heat and alternate between that and the cool setting to cause less heat damage and avoid removing too much moisture from the hair.
- If you have thick hair, look for a blow dryer with a higher wattage (like 1875W) as these will often dry your hair faster.
- Look for tourmaline and ceramic blow dryers for smoother results.
- Finish off with the cool setting to seal your hair cuticle and set your style.

Hooded Dryer:

- Keep it on medium setting as the highest setting will start to dry out your hair.
- Try wearing a satin cap to trap the heat and dry the hair faster in a shorter period of time.

Flat Iron:

- Only use a flat iron that has a temperature gauge so that you know exactly how much heat you are using. I rarely go above 400 degrees.
- When flat ironing hair, focus more on the roots and less on the ends as they are more fragile.
- Never flat iron dirty hair, make sure it is freshly washed and conditioned.
- Do not go over each strand more than twice.
- Purchase a flat iron that is ceramic or tourmaline.
- Always make sure your flat iron is clean.

Pressing Comb:

- Honestly this is a tool of the past and that's where it should stay unless you are a licensed professional.

Curling Iron:

- Be sure to use one with a temperature gauge, and don't hold the curling iron on your hair too long.

Diffuser:

- ✦ This blow dryer attachment reduces frizz that natural hair often experiences when air drying.
- ✦ Reduces heat damage to hair and makes curls pop!
- ✦ Adds volume and shine.

So is heat really bad for my hair?

Not all heat! For example, a hooded dryer used during the deep conditioning process is actually beneficial for your hair. This method of indirect heat allows the hair cuticle to open and absorb the moisture without harming the hair.

How often can I flat iron my hair?

Everyone's hair is different in how much heat it can handle. As a rule of thumb, once your hair has been flat ironed do not try to "touch it up" every day. Flat ironing your hair everyday will cause heat damage and permanently straighten those natural curls. I try to get two weeks out of my flat iron.

For maximum growth I would only flat iron once a month, if that. We have both seen the most hair growth when we've gone at least three months with no heat. If you miss straight hair that much, opt for a straight wig or weave.

Can heat damage be reversed?

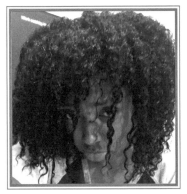

When you find someone who has reversed heat damage, send them our way! At one point my hair was severely damaged from using the flat iron way too much. I attempted to repair it with several protein and deep conditioner treatments and had no luck. The more heat you use the more you alter the protein structure of the hair, which changes how your curls look. You will find that some naturals who wear weaves regularly and flat iron their "leave out" have heat damage in certain parts of their hair. You can use treatments to strengthen and condition the hair but ultimately once that hair is heat damaged, it will not revert back. Heat damage doesn't bother some naturals. But if you are set on avoiding heat damage, then you need to watch how much heat you apply to your hair. Victoria still has a few strands of her hair that are heat damaged, but they don't bother her.

How hot is too hot?

My best rule of thumb is to stay under 380°F if you can. Some textures are harder to straighten than other textures so keep in mind if you have major shrinkage you might need more heat than someone with a looser curl pattern. If you are flat ironing try to only go over each section one good time.

Is it safe to mix permanent dyes and heat on natural hair?

Heat and chemicals are the only two things that can permanently alter the structure of hair. It is very important to deep condition the hair regularly. Use products made for color treated hair. If you have color treated hair, you will want to avoid heat even more. Some people bleach their hair and flat iron it successfully without major breakage. There is major hair maintenance involved with color treated hair. We both experienced breakage from coloring our hair so we always recommend staying away from permanent hair color.

Listen, we don't want you to be scared to use heat. Just remember to use everything in moderation. Our hair thrives best in it's natural state.

Look at what no heat can do for your hair!

Moisture—Heat = GROWTH!

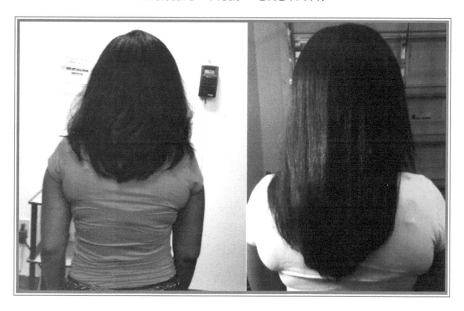

6 months NO HEAT!

Some Additional Tips:

- **ALWAYS** deep condition your hair before applying heat to the hair.
- Air-drying is really the healthiest method for drying your hair.
- Try to use one heat source. For example, if you are going to flat iron your hair, let it air-dry overnight then flat iron it the next day.
- Try taking a break from heat in 3-6 month increments. This will keep your hair strong and healthy.

WINTER HAIR CARE VS. SUMMER HAIR CARE

Your hair care needs may change based on the time of year. Does it seem like your hair is extra dry in the winter or that your hair seems to thrive in the summer? The outside environment does affect your hair and the main seasons we want to focus on are winter and summer.

Winter Hair Care

Depending on where you live, winter may be harsher for some naturals. If you're a natural that lives in Florida, you will have a different winter hair care regimen than someone who lives in New York.

To keep it simple, here's a few **winter tips**:

- Since most winter wardrobes consist of sweaters, scarves and hats, it's important to remember to keep your hair from rubbing against any rough fabric. It is easy for your hair to get snagged on your favorite sweater. Certain hats can also dry your hair out. Try a satin lined hat. Remember your hair needs to be spoiled!
- Since hair seems much drier in the winter, add an extra deep conditioning session to keep your hair moisturized.
- Use heavier creams to lock in moisture. If you normally use a liquid leave-in conditioner or daily moisturizer, try a cream based product.
- This is the perfect time to wear straighter styles since there isn't as much humidity. Your straight style will last much longer. (But don't overdo the use of heat).
- Baby your ends! Focus your moisturizing on the ends of your hair. They are the oldest part of your hair. Make sure to seal the moisture in with a light oil.

- Tuck your ends if possible with styles such as buns, wigs or weaves.
- Protective Style. This is the perfect time for the big curly long weaves we all love. You know the styles that are too hot to wear during the summer. Twists and buns are also great options to keep your hair off your shoulders.
- To all my wash and go ladies: Try to avoid leaving the house with wet hair in the cold weather.

Summer Hair Care

For most naturals, this is the best time of year to play and experiment with your hair. Flaunt your wash and go in the summer sun! However, this is the time of year where humidity is a bit higher so you can see an increase in frizz.

To keep it simple, here's a few **summer tips**:

- Always stay hydrated by drinking lots of water.
- If you are wearing a wash and go, keep your hair moist even if you have to carry around a spray bottle and spritz once or twice a day. I personally mix aloe vera gel in my spray bottle with water for extra nutrients.
- Try to avoid wearing straight hair too much. Those hours spent flat ironing your hair won't matter soon as you leave the house and your hair hits that humidity.
- Use anti-frizz sprays or serums to reduce frizz.
- Everyone's hair is different but try adding in an extra cowash session during the week.
- **ALWAYS** clarify and deep condition your hair after going swimming. Chlorine and salt water can be very damaging to your hair. It helps to saturate your hair with water and conditioner before you get in the pool so that your hair soaks up less chlorine.
- Shea butter is one of the best products all year around. If it's too thick and hard for you, try whipped shea butter. Thank us later!

CHARTING YOUR HAIR GROWTH

One of the biggest complaints we hear from naturals is that their hair isn't growing. The truth is your hair is growing. The problem is that either you are not retaining your hair length or you are not noticing your hair growth. Here's our top tips for charting your hair growth.

Take pictures of your hair every three months. It doesn't matter if you think your hair has not grown. Pictures don't lie. Start today by taking a picture of your hair. In three months take another picture. Seeing growth will motivate you to continue taking care of your hair.

Set hair goals. We are firm believers that what you think will happen will eventually happen. Speak positive and believe your hair is growing and watch it grow. Hold yourself accountable.

Expect setbacks. Trust us. It's normal to fall off of your hair regimen. Life happens. You can always get right back on it. Don't give up. It took us years to perfect our hair care regimen and actually learn to take care of our hair.

Show off your progress! Growing your hair is a big deal and don't let anybody tell you otherwise. Post progress pictures on Instagram and Facebook. It inspires other naturals in more ways than you know. At the very end of this book you will find your very own personal hair growth chart. Rip it out and hang it up!

CHAPTER 3

The Conservative Natural

In our opinion, there are two types of naturals. Desiree and I just happen to be completely opposites when it comes to our natural hair. I'm the cautious, conservative one who refuses to leave the house with a wash and go or big chop my hair. Desiree, is the bold, adventurous one who big chopped twice without giving it a second thought. For all my ladies like her the next chapter was written just for you.

In this section, we'll go over styles and tips for the ladies who aren't quite ready to walk out the door with the big natural hair.

Side note: There's nothing wrong with being either natural. It's all about comfort. There is a natural style for every occasion. For example, if you have an important corporate job interview, you might want to opt for a sleek natural bun. On the other hand, if you're going out on a date, you might want a voluminous, sexy twist out or wash and go. Our favorite part of being natural is the versatility. You can literally create whatever style you want on your natural hair.

So for all my conservative naturals, let's explore some style options.

WIGS

Wigs are my absolute favorite protective style and I wear wigs a LOT.

Why do I wear wigs so much?

You can achieve many different looks (curly, wavy or straight). Wigs work for me and I retain a lot of my hair length.

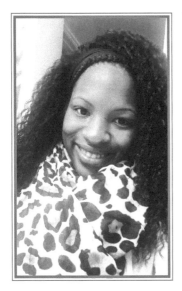

The biggest benefit of wigs is that you can take it off daily and moisturize your hair. If you've been reading through this book so far you will hear us repeat how important moisturizing is to growing and retaining your hair length.

I take my wig off every night and moisturize my natural hair. I do not comb my hair at all. With most of my wigs, my natural hair is in 8 big twists underneath. I do not untwist or mess with the twists until wash day. This means that if I wear my wig daily for about a month and I wash my hair weekly, I only comb my hair about 4 times that month. I'm not pulling at my hair or causing any manipulation to my hair on a daily basis. I'm leaving it alone. This has literally helped me grow my hair longer than it has ever been.

Here's my top wig wearing tips:

Don't spend a ton of money on wigs. There are plenty of cheap $20-$30 wigs that are synthetic hair and will last you at least a month with proper care of the wig. (Amazon has some great wig options). Curly synthetic hair tends to actually blend well with our natural hair texture.

It's important to note, I do invest in quality hair extensions as well. I don't mind spending the money because I know the extensions will last me multiple uses.

Invest in rollers, flexi-rods, or perm rods. These items will help blend your leave out with curly wigs.

With natural hair, I stay away from straight wigs unless it is a full wig.

Take the wig combs out of your wig to avoid causing tension around your edges. I use bobby pins to secure my wig.

Take care of your wigs to get them to last longer. Most wigs come with care instructions. I typically cowash my wig and hang it to dry.

KNOW WHEN TO THROW THE WIG AWAY. We want you ladies to look absolutely beautiful so if your wig is matted or is ridiculously frizzy, get rid of it.

Please remember to moisturize your natural hair underneath the wig. Dry hair will split and you will end up having to trim your hair more often.

SEW INS

When I first went natural I wore a lot of sew ins. It made me feel good knowing I didn't have to worry about someone pulling my wig off.

Sew ins make us feel like the hair is growing out of our scalp.

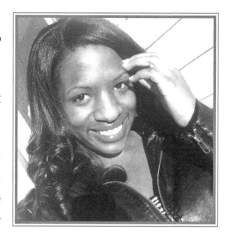

My only problem with my sew ins was that I ended up with heat damage in the top section of my hair. You know where you have that little bit of "leave out" hair that you blend to hide the tracks. Mind you I've had some flawless sew ins.

My biggest downfall was not moisturizing my hair underneath my sew ins. With my Brazilian weave I didn't want to put oil on my hair underneath and risk the weave looking greasy. So I ignored my natural hair underneath. All I was worried about was did the weave look good.

After noticing extreme dryness and split ends, I stopped wearing sew ins and moved on over to wigs.

If you absolutely have to have your sew in, make sure you find a way to moisturize your hair. Try to limit the use of heat on your leave out. Find extensions that will blend easily with your natural hair.

BUNS/UPDOS

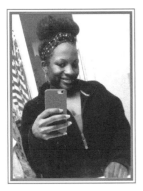

Buns are cute and chic ways to style your hair. Now that my hair is longer, I can make full buns with just my own hair. When my hair was shorter I would add some synthetic braiding hair to my bun to make it fuller.

Here's some tips when wearing your hair up:

Do not pull your hair too tight. Pulling your hair back too tight causes stress on your edges.

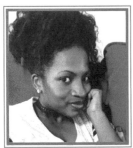

Tuck your ends if possible. But don't be afraid of putting a failed twist out up either. It's one of my favorite looks.

Add hair accessories to spice up your look.

*Try not to wear your bun in the same position. Alternate a high bun or low bun.

BRAIDS AND TWISTS

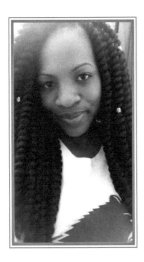

So for one year when I was in high school I wore braids for a whole year. Not the same braids. But I literally took my braids out on a Friday and put new braids in the next day. I got a ton of new growth but my hair ended up extremely dry and my ends split. By time I gave my hair a break I needed a major trim. Needless to say, I didn't keep much of that length. Moral of the story: Don't wear braids or twists too often.

When I wear box braids now, I moisturize my hair as much as possible. I don't care if that means my braids get a little frizzy. Gel or a pomade will help keep your braids looking as neat as possible.

Massage and oil your scalp. You don't want to clog your pores so I wouldn't suggest doing this everyday. It's best to apply a light oil to your scalp and massage it in a few times a week.

Also, I spray my braids with water or let the steam from the shower give them a little moisture.

I never pull my braids back too tight. Braids can be harsh on your edges. So give your edges a break. If you want to wear your braids up make sure it's loose.

MY FINAL TIP: EXPERIMENT WITH DIFFERENT TYPES OF CURLS

It's ok to be a little conservative. You can still have fun with your curls. You can create just about any curl with the right products and tools.

When it comes to products, look for twisting creams or holding gels that will give you just the right amount of hold. Also, rubbing a little oil through your hair as you take down rollers or any of these styles will help cut down on the frizz.

Here's some of my favorite styling tools:

- Perm rods—this will give you that soft curly look
- Curlformers—these will give you a spiral curl
- Rollers—the smaller the roller, the tighter the curl

Other Methods to Create Curls or Waves:

- Flat twists
- Bantu knots
- Braids
- Two strand twists

Ladies, you will have many failed hairstyles. It doesn't mean you give up. With practice comes perfection. Sometimes I have to redo a simple bun. It happens. The key is to never stop trying. Learn to love the process and you will get great results.

CHAPTER 4

The Bold Natural

Being able to freely wear their curls is one of the main reasons why women go natural. A "Bold Natural" is a woman who prefers to rock her curls in its natural state or with very low manipulation. Victoria gets the luxury of being versatile but if you're like me your scalp don't play when it comes to wigs, weave or synthetic hair for braids. I have tried several different options with no luck, so I just rock my curls. There are still a variety of styling options that we can choose. I'll give you a few style ideas!

FROHAWKS

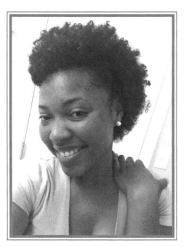

When I first went natural I wasn't comfortable wearing my "mini-fro" and I thought I looked like a boy. I started experimenting with my hair and that is when I discovered the "Frohawk". Through trial and error I perfected this style and I clung to it for like the first year of my big chop.

I'm not going to lie, when I first went natural I had no idea what I was doing or what products to use. The frohawk was super quick and convenient but my hair was extremely dry. It took me quite some time to learn about the LOC method for retaining moisture and which products were best for my hair. Back when I first went natural there were not nearly as many natural hair products on the market to help me achieve this style as there are today. This hairstyle is super easy but don't get lazy and just spray your hair with water and go. Your hair needs to be thoroughly moisturized.

Tip: Use bobby pins or small clamps to pin your hair up on one side or both sides to achieve this look. If you want it to look more natural you don't have to add gel or edge control but I do.

Do not pull your hair too tight when you pin up your hair. You do not want to stress your edges.

BANTU KNOTS

After about a year I was more confident with my hair length and wanted to try something new. That's when I discovered "Bantu Knots" on YouTube. This is one of my favorites because it results in such a pretty curl. After a year, I had grown a ton of thick and long hair so this was a style that definitely took more time.

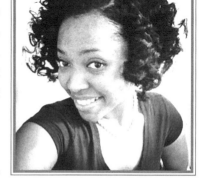

You have the option to do this on wet or dry hair. If you do it on dry hair make sure to use some type leave-in conditioner or a twist cream to lightly moisturize your hair so that the curls will dry and stay in place. Some naturals wear the bantu knots themselves and some untwist them. I have also seen a combination of both but I haven't had the courage to leave the house in just knots lol!

Tips:

If your knots don't stay in place by just wrapping them, you can use bobby pins or ponytail holders.

Let the bantu knots dry at least a day and a half for the best results. If you unwrap them too soon they will still be wet which will result in frizzy and droopy curls. Apply oil to your hands before unwrapping your knots.

The size of the bantu knot will determine the size of the curl. The smaller your knots are the tighter your curls will be. Try bigger knots for larger curls and bounce!

TWIST OUTS

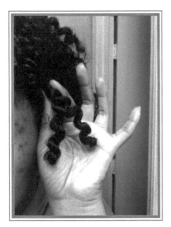

Twist outs are pretty much the go to for naturals since it produces the best curl definition. I would be lying if I said this is a favorite. For me this style takes a little too long because I have **SUPER** thick, stubborn hair.

You have the option of doing braids, two strand or three strand twists. The key to this hairstyle is finding a good combination of products and taking your time for ideal results. From my experience twist outs work better on longer hair. I never did a twist out when I did my first big chop and since my second big chop I don't use this style too often. Hopefully as this journey continues I'll experiment more! But I do have a few tips if you plan to try a twist out.

Tips:

- Give your hair a full day or two to let the twist dry or sit under the dryer. If you untwist them while they are partially wet you will get tons of frizz and your curls won't last. Make sure to sleep in a bonnet to keep them in place.
- Apply oil to your hands to untwist and separate your twists to avoid frizz.
- Use a pick comb to separate it at the roots and give your twist out more volume.

PINEAPPLE PONYTAIL

Now this is another favorite of mine because it's super easy. After this second big chop, my hair finally reached a length long enough so that I can wear this style again. This is the perfect option for an old twist out or wash and go when you need your hair to last a few more days. It also works great on freshly wet hair as the hair is easier to manipulate. I usually wear my wash and go's down but I resort to this when it gets too hot and I want my hair out of my face!

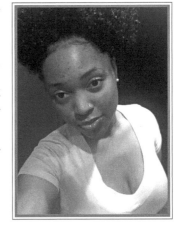

Tips:

- Make sure you LOC or LCO (this style dries out quickly) and pull your hair gently to prevent breakage.
- If you can gel it down and mold the style with your hands, do so. The less manipulation the better.
- To make those edges look sleek, use some gel, edge control and a brush. I suggest getting an edge brush as it's able to manipulate your edges much better!

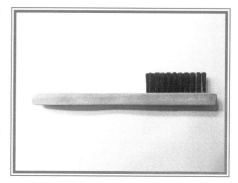

WASH AND GO

I had to save the best for last in my opinion. From when I first went natural until now I still love a quick wash and go! You should part your hair in sections and perform the LCO or LOC method on your hair to retain moisture. Some people apply products with their hands but I have found the secret to making your curls pop is to use a Denman brush as it smooths the hair out while clumping your curls beautifully. Because I'm so busy these days, my hands usually do the trick and I'm fine with how it looks.

Tips:

- Use a diffuser to dry your hair faster, reduce frizz and preserve your curls before you leave the house.
- You can wear cute headbands to give your wash and go some life.
- Wear your wash and go in different styles such as middle part, side part, or even half up and half down.
- For super defined curls you can use a gel to clump your curls. In my opinion **Eco Styler Black Castor and Flaxseed Oil Gel** is the equivalent of gold for curl definition and frizz reduction!

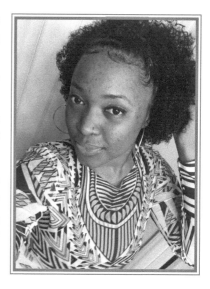

Spritz your hair once or twice a day with a water, conditioner, oil mix to retain moisture since your hair can dry out fast!

Final tip: Some of these styles require more maintenance than others but always remember to properly moisturize and seal your hair. To be honest, I wasn't comfortable when I cut my hair the first or second time. Through trial and error I learned what looked cute on me and what worked best for my hair. Don't feel like you have to hide your hair just because you don't like your curls. I promise with some practice and the right products you will grow to love your curls.

Ultimately, I want all of you to grow to love your curls no matter the length or pattern!

CHAPTER 5

Natural Hair on a Budget

Don't go broke trying to buy every new product you see. There's great natural hair products and styles for every budget.

If you're on a budget, below are some great tips for you to get the most out of your hair growth journey:

BUY SAMPLE SIZES WHEN TRYING NEW PRODUCTS.

Most beauty supply stores and hair stores offer sample sizes of different hair products. Before you buy the big bottle of a new conditioner, try the smaller size to make sure it works for your hair. Also, check different hair product websites. They often sell trial size or sample sets of their products. Sometimes you might even get a few free samples.

KNOW WHEN TO SAVE AND KNOW WHEN TO SPLURGE.

Save and opt for a cheaper shampoo. A little shampoo goes a long way. Splurge on your deep conditioners. This is what your hair really needs.

TRY PRODUCTS THAT DOUBLE IN USE.

Some products double as a gentle cleanser and conditioner. Keep your regimen simple and add on slowly. You can also try using your leave-in conditioner as your daily moisturizer as well.

TAKE A LOOK AROUND YOUR KITCHEN.

There are all sorts of things in your kitchen that you can use in your hair. Bananas, eggs, mayonnaise, olive oil and honey are just a few items that work wonders for the hair.

KNOW THE BASICS OF WHAT YOU NEED IN YOUR HAIR REGIMEN.

The **basics** are:

- Shampoo
- Deep conditioner
- Leave-in conditioner/Daily moisturizer
- Oil
- Styler (only if you do styles like wash and go's)

Here are some of our favorite budget friendly brands:

- Herbal Essence
- Aussie
- VO5
- Tresemme
- Ecostyler
- Suave
- Organix
- Creme of Nature

CONDITIONING YOUR HAIR ON A BUDGET

You can still condition your hair successfully when on a budget. Try adding oils to cheap conditioners for a deeper conditioning.

You can still find a way to add heat to your deep conditioning without a hooded dryer. If you don't have a dryer to sit under, take a towel and put it in the dryer while you wash your hair. Once you apply your deep conditioner, apply a plastic cap or plastic bag to the hair and wrap the hot towel around the plastic cap. Another option is to do some jumping jacks or crunches while you your deep conditioner is in. Generating body heat will also help open your hair cuticles.

When it comes to choosing an oil for your hair, look for a product that is a mixture of oils. That way you don't have to buy a lot of separate oils.

STYLING YOUR HAIR ON A BUDGET

Choose cheaper protective styles. Instead of spending hundreds of dollars on weave bundles, opt for cheaper, synthetic weaves. Some of my best looks are using $20 wigs. Never underestimate the use of bobby pins to achieve awesome looks. Use YouTube. There are tons of natural hair tutorials. Invest in hair accessories. Scarves and headbands can turn your plain bun into a cute chic style.

LASTLY, MY BIGGEST PIECE OF ADVICE WHEN ON A BUDGET IS TO MAKE A PLAN.

Decide to buy one new hair product a month until you have everything you need. Don't feel pressured to buy a product just because it's popular or works for everyone else. Listen to your hair.

As we discussed in Chapter 2, the key to getting the most out of your hair regimen is to know what products and tools you already have.

We do not want you to think that you have to spends tons of money to grow your hair. One of my many mistakes was buying too many products at one time. Some of those products just ended up collecting dust.

CHAPTER 6

Fitness and Diet for Naturals

What's fitness and diet got to do with hair growth? You'd be surprised to find how much a little diet improvement and fitness will benefit your hair. Not only will your hair benefit from you living a healthy hairstyle, but your body will love you for it.

A known stereotype for black women is that we avoid working out because we don't want to ruin our hair. I'm guilty of it. Especially when I was relaxed and I just got my hair done. I stayed far away from anything that would make me sweat. When I went natural, one of the perks I noticed right away was that since my hair wasn't straight anymore I didn't have to worry about "sweating my hair out".

Now, I set my hair around my fitness routine and make my hairstyles workout friendly.

We will give you a few hair options in this chapter if you want to lead an active lifestyle.

Let's cover fitness first and then we'll tackle diet.

FITNESS

So when's the best time to workout?

That's actually up to you. There are pros and cons to working out first thing in the morning before you start your day and pros and cons to working out at the end of your day. I find it easier to do it first thing in the morning.

Morning Workouts

Pros

- You get it done and out the way
- Some people believe working out first thing in the morning on an empty stomach is better for losing weight
- You force yourself to wake up earlier
- By time you are done working out you are wide awake and energized

Cons

- You may sweat out certain hairstyles before day starts
- You have to wake up earlier

Evening Workouts

Pros

- Your hair has time to set overnight
- Perfect way to wind down after a long day
- Don't have to worry about being late for work

Cons

- You may be tired at the end of the day and less likely to follow through with your workout
- If something comes up unexpectedly you will have to sacrifice your workout

Style Options for Naturals with an Active Lifestyle

- Braids
- Twists
- Wigs
- Crotchet braids
- Updos
- Wash and go

Hair Maintenance Tips

- Cowash more often—sweat can build up in your hair and dry it out.
- Plan your workouts and coordinate your hairstyles. If you have straight hair at the beginning of the week, do your lighter workouts. As the week progresses, do your more intense workouts and start to wear your hair up.

Naturals that Wear Their Hair Straight

- Make sure you aren't tempted to re-straighten your hair too often.
- If your roots are really wet after working out you can blow dry the roots only—try using the cool setting.
- Try large rollers to stretch the hair without having to use heat.
- Try wrapping hair during your workout and leave your hair wrapped until hair is completely dry from any sweat.
- Don't be afraid of not having bone straight hair.

Now that we've gotten the exercise part out the way, let's cover diet.

DIET

A lot of people forget that your diet is beneficial to hair growth. I'm no dietitian but I've seen the most growth when I had a healthier diet. Check this out!

WATER! WATER! WATER!

- I know some of you may not be a fan of water. I mean it has no taste so it's not the most appetizing. Hydrated hair grows. You have to hydrate the hair from the inside out.
- One thing I do remember from my high school biology class is that water is responsible for a lot! It hydrates the body, flushes out toxins, provides vitamins/minerals, and controls cell health/reproduction which is what grows your hair.

Protein

- Since your hair is made up of protein it makes perfect sense for your diet to consist of a healthy amount of protein to maintain cell production.
- Protein is responsible for repair and growth so you must include the right amount in your diet.
- Focus on good proteins like eggs, tuna, lean chicken, beans and nuts.

Vitamins/Minerals

- **Vitamin A**—Your scalp uses this to produce sebum which lubricates the hair roots and prevents scalp from getting dry. (Found in spinach, carrots, apricots, peaches, meat, dairy, etc.)
- **Vitamin B6**—Contributes to blood circulation and cell-building. (Found in liver, whole grains, eggs, veggies, etc.)
- **Vitamin B12**—Important nutrient in growth and strength of hair. (Found in chicken, eggs, milk, fish, bananas, sunflower seeds, etc.)
- **Biotin**—Enhances growth, thickens hair shaft, lessens hair loss. (Found in eggs, dairy, liver, etc.)
- **Vitamin C**—Contributes to production of red blood cells. (Found in strawberries, pineapples, kiwi, citrus fruits, tomatoes, etc.)
- **Vitamin E**—Essential for good blood circulation, which feeds the hair follicles (where your hair grows from) and keeps them healthy. (Found in olive oil, canola oil, soybeans, nuts, seeds, dried beans, etc.)
- **Inositol**—Maintains healthy membranes that make up hair. (Found in whole grains, citrus, fruit, bananas, brown rice, nuts, most veggies, liver, etc.)
- **Iron**—Contributes to the production of red blood cells. (Found in spinach, broccoli, lean beef, dark meat, chicken, turkey, etc.)
- **Niacin**—Helps circulation in scalp to promote hair growth. (Found in fish, poultry, meat, wheat germ, etc.)
- **Vitamin B5**—Located in most shampoos and promotes healthy hair growth. (Found in whole grains, eggs, beef, veggies, beans, pork, saltwater fish, whole rye flour, whole wheat flour)
- **Zinc**—Contributes to the function of hair follicles so hair can grow properly. (Found in seafood, poultry, whole grains, nuts, brewer's yeast, etc.)

*Majority of these vitamins and minerals can be found in a good **multivitamin** if you are unable to get all of them on a daily basis from food alone. However, it is best to create a healthy diet that is composed of them. A lot of sugars and fatty foods do not contain these vitamins and minerals which means that you are not getting the proper nutrients to help grow your hair!*

CHAPTER 7

Products to Try

Here are some of our favorite products by category. Remember this list doesn't cover all of the awesome hair products out there. This list is just to give you ladies some suggestions.

This list only includes products we have actually tried.

Shampoos

- Creme of Nature Argan Oil Shampoo
- ORS Aloe Shampoo (use only for clarifying your hair)
- SheaMoisture Jamaican Black Castor Oil Strengthen, Grow & Restore Shampoo
- TGIN Moisture Rich Sulfate Free Shampoo
- SheaMoisture Raw Shea Butter Moisture Retention Shampoo
- Mielle Organics Babassu Oil Conditioning Sulfate-Free Shampoo

Leave-in Conditioners

- Mielle Organics Peony Leave-in
- Creme of Nature Argan Oil 7-in-1 Leave-in
- Karen's Body Beautiful Sweet Ambrosia Leave-in
- Carol's Daughter Sacred Tiare Leave-In
- Miss Jessie's Original Leave-in

Conditioners

- As I Am Coconut CoWash Cleansing Conditioner

- Herbal Essence Hello Hydration Moisturizing Conditioner
- Hair One Hair Cleanser & Conditioner
- Aussie Total Miracle 7N1 Conditioner
- Aussie 3 Minute Miracle
- Aussie Mega Moist Conditioner
- Tresemme Moisture Rich Conditioner
- Trader Joe's Nourish Spa Conditioner
- TGIN Triple Moisture Replenishing Conditioner

Deep Conditioners

- Creme of Nature Argan Oil Intensive Conditioning Treatment
- Eden BodyWorks Jojoba Monoi Natural Deep Conditioner
- Mielle Organics Babassu Oil Mint Deep Conditioner
- ORS Replenishing Deep Conditioner
- TGIN Honey Miracle Mask
- Carol's Daughter Hair Milk Curl-Defining Moisture Mask
- Hair One Hair Masque with Olive Oil
- SheaMoisture Jamaican Black Castor Oil Strengthen, Grow & Restore Treatment Mask
- Macadamia Oil Deep Repair Mask
- SheaMoisture Raw Shea Butter Deep Treatment Masque
- Camille Rose Naturals Algae Renew Deep Conditioner

Protein Treatments

- ORS Hair Mayonnaise Treatment
- Palmer's Coconut Oil Deep Conditioning Protein Pack
- Nutress Hair Moisturizing Protein Pack

Daily Moisturizers

- TGIN Butter Cream Daily Moisturizer
- SheaMoisture Coconut & Hibiscus Curl Milk `

Stylers/Gels

- Jane Carter Solution Wrap & Roll
- Ecostyler Gels
- Camille Rose Naturals Almond Jai Twisting Butter

- ORS Olive Oil Smooth-N-Hold Pudding
- Miss Jessie's Pillow Soft Curls
- Miss Jessie's Curly Pudding

Pomades/Butters

- Jane Carter Nourish and Shine Hair Butter
- Design Essentials Sleek Max Edge Control

Heat Protectants

- CHI Silk Infusion
- Tresemme Heat Tamer Leave-In Spray
- Aussie Hair Insurance Heat Protecting Shine Spray

Take Away

We are just two girls who decided years ago that we wanted to take a different journey with our hair. Through trial and error we found many things that worked for us. Keep in mind that we hit just as many roadblocks. There were times when we wanted to throw in the towel but we thought about how far we came and realized that giving up wasn't an option. When we finally learned what to do, we wanted to share it with others. Your journey will definitely be different from the next girl but don't let that deter you. There are so many girls who have long, beautiful hair including ourselves and we want that for you too. We are very passionate about growing healthy hair. This is not a lengthy book on natural hair. We just wanted to scratch the surface to help get you started. This is your personal guide to hold onto and reference as often as you need. We hope that you enjoyed our goddess guide and we want to hear from you! Tell us your hair stories and share some of your experiences. We are already working on our next big project to help educate and enhance your natural hair experience. Stay tuned!

In the meantime, connect with us via email, Facebook or Instagram!

THE CURL GODDESS GUIDE

FACEBOOK

Curl Goddess Girls

EMAIL

curlgoddessgirls@gmail.com

Instagram

Desiree Davis - Melanin.Muze
Victoria Russell - Victorias_hair_corner

About the Authors

DESIREE DAVIS

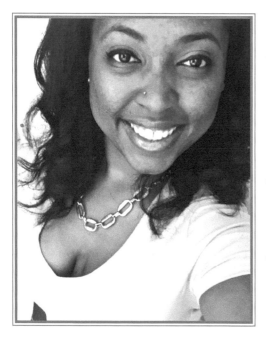

Desiree is an aspiring entrepreneur who began her natural hair journey in 2010 with a big chop. After graduating from The University of North Carolina Greensboro, she began working full time. In order to pursue her real passion and talent as an artist, she left her full-time job to become a full-time artist. She has had the honor of presenting her art to various celebrities such as: Trent Shelton, Pascale Rowe (Ms. Bling Miami), Ming Lee and Jermell Charlo. By November 2016, she had her first art show. Natural hair was something she continued to grow passionate about which led to her second big chop in 2016. Her goal was to embark on a healthier hair growth journey. Born in California, this free spirit likes to travel and read in her spare time while being a full-time mommy to her dog Khloe.

VICTORIA RUSSELL

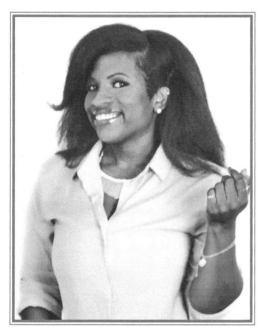

Victoria is also an aspiring entrepreneur who began her natural hair journey in 2012 when she transitioned from relaxed hair to natural hair during her last year of undergraduate studies at The University of North Carolina Greensboro. Upon graduation, she continued her studies through an online graduate degree program with Liberty University, while working full-time for the City of Raleigh. During this time, she continued to study and experiment with natural hair care. After she received her MBA in 2014, she began to dedicate more time to studying and practicing techniques to grow and retain natural hair. Victoria was born and raised in Pennsylvania and has currently resided in North Carolina for the past nine years. She is most recently the proud mother of a ten month old beautiful baby girl, Mikaela.

My Curl Goddess Hair Growth Journey

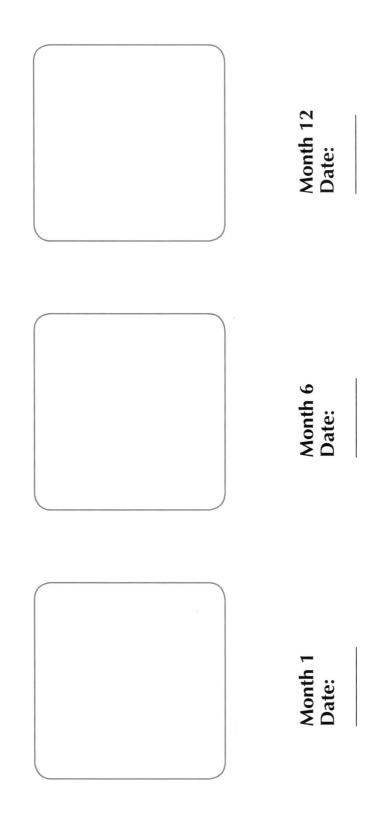

Month 1
Date: _____

Month 6
Date: _____

Month 12
Date: _____

MY HAIR PRODUCT INVENTORY

Write each product you already have and decide if you will keep it on not. This step will help you with the next page.

Shampoos: _____
_____
_____
_____
_____
_____
_____

Conditioners: _____
_____
_____
_____
_____
_____
_____

Stylers/Oils: _____
_____
_____
_____
_____
_____
_____

What Products I Need: _____
_____
_____
_____
_____
_____

MY PERSONAL HAIR REGIMEN

Here you should list the products you will use regularly. Update it when your hair needs a change or you find a product you like better. Having a great set of hair product staples takes the guessing game out of creating your perfect regimen.

My Favorite Shampoos/Cleansers: _____

_____

_____

_____

_____

_____

My Favorite Conditioners: _____

_____

_____

_____

_____

_____

_____

My Favorite Daily Moisturizers: _____

_____

_____

_____

_____

_____

_____

My Favorite Styling Products: _____

_____

_____

_____

_____

_____

_____

My Favorite Oils: _____

_____

_____

_____

_____

_____

SOURCES

Donaldson, Chris-Tia. Thank God I'm Natural: The Ultimate Guide to Caring for and Maintaining Natural Hair. Chicago: TgiNesis, 2014. Print.

D'Souza, P., & Rathi, S. (2015). Shampoo and conditioners: What a dermatologist should know? *Indian Journal of Dermatology, 60*(3), 248-254. doi:http://dx.doi.org. ezproxy.liberty.edu/10.4103/0019-5154.156355

Evans, Trefor A., Ph.D. "Beating the Damaging Effects of Heat on Hair." *Cosmetics & Toiletries*, T.A Evans Inc, 4 June 2015. Web. 18 Mar. 2017.

Madnani, Nina, and Kaleem Khan. "Hair cosmetics." *Indian Journal of Dermatology, Venereology and Leprology,* vol. 79, no. 5, 2013, p. 654. *General OneFile,* ezproxy.liberty.edu/login?url=http://go.galegroup.com.ezproxy.liberty.edu/ps/i. do?p=ITOF&sw=w&u=vic_liberty&v=2.1&it=r?7id=GALE%7CA341738088&sid=su mmon&asid=0dd3771219885b9e5607f2728a94a7016. Accessed 25 June 2017.

ProgressiveHealth. "16 Vitamin Deficiencies That Lead to Hair Loss." *HealDove*. HealDove, 10 June 2015. Web. 24 Apr. 2017.

Strehlow, Anne T. "Other Traits." *Understanding Genetics*. The Tech Museum of Innovation, 26 Apr. 2005. Web. 13 Mar. 2017.

CPSIA information can be obtained
at www.ICGtesting.com
Printed in the USA
LVHW071040200120
644154LV00004B/84